CW01455065

Renal Diet Cookbook for Beginners

The Best Guide with Simple Recipes to Learn How to Prepare Delicious Dishes for Kidney Disease Diet

By Elizabeth Lopez

© **Copyright 2021 by (Elizabeth Lopez)- All rights reserved.**

This document is geared towards providing exact and reliable information regarding the topic and issue covered. The publication is sold with the idea that the publisher is not required to render accounting, officially permitted or otherwise qualified services. If advice is necessary, legal, or professional, a practiced individual in the profession should be ordered.From a Declaration of Principles which was accepted and approved equally by a Committee of the American Bar Association and a Committee of Publishers and Associations. In no way is it legal to reproduce, duplicate, or transmit any part of this document in either electronic means or printed format. The recording of this publication is strictly prohibited. Any storage of this document is not allowed unless with written permission from the publisher. All rights reserved. The information provided herein is stated to be truthful and consistent. In terms of inattention or otherwise, any liability, by any usage or abuse of any policies, processes, or Instructions contained within is the recipient reader's solitary and utter responsibility. Under no circumstances will any legal responsibility or blame be held against the publisher for reparation, damages, or monetary loss due to the information herein, either directly or indirectly. Respective authors own all copyrights not held by the publisher. The information herein is offered for informational purposes solely and is universal as so. The presentation of the information is without a contract or any guarantee assurance. The trademarks used are without any consent. The publication of the trademark is without permission or backing by the trademark owner. All trademarks and brands within this book are for clarifying purposes only and are owned by the owners themselves, not affiliated with this document.

Sommario

Introduction

This cookbook, is designed and written for beginners, for people who suffer from kidney disease, want to maintain optimal health levels by cooking healthy, unrefined, tasty and above all simple foods.

That's because in chronic kidney disease (CKD) outcomes, diet plays a critical role. In people with end-stage renal

end-stage renal disease (ESRD), protein-energy wasting and inflammation are among the leading risk factors for death. In people with mild to moderate levels of kidney failure, diet can be directly or indirectly linked scientifically to key components of CKD treatment, including blood pressure regulation and management of dyslipidemia, diabetes.

Before we begin I want to give you a very important piece of advice and that is to minimize the consumption of salt and potassium, which act negatively on the kidneys that already sick cannot dispose of them in the best way creating other serious disorders.

But now let's start with the recipes....

Chapter 1: Kidney friendly Renal Diet Breakfast Recipes

1. Lemon Apple Honey Smoothie

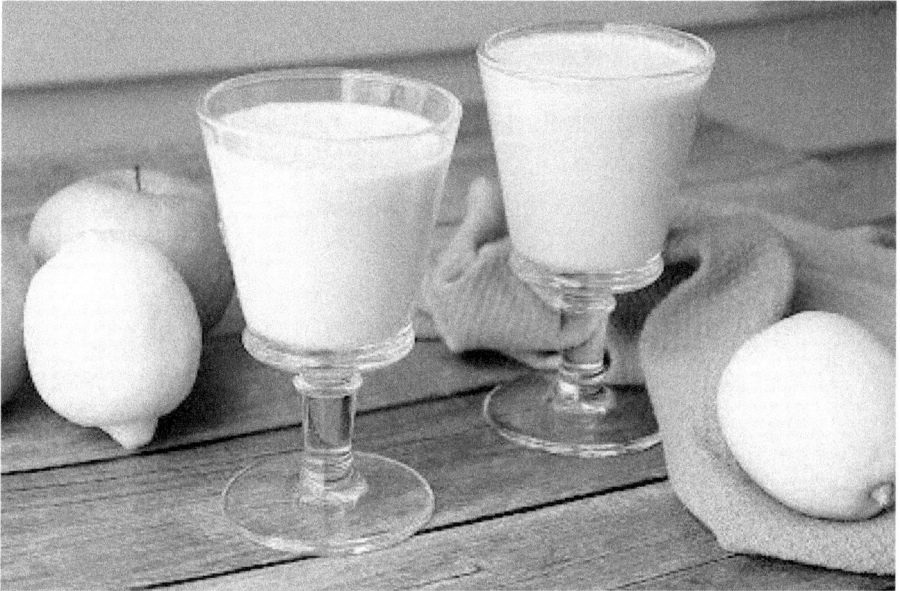

|Calories:170 | Total time: 5min | Servings: 4 | Difficulty: Easy

Ingredients

- Lemon juice, 1/4 cup

- Apple juice, 1/2 cup

- Peeled and cored apple, 1

- 1 banana

- Honey, 2-3 teaspoons

- Vanilla frozen yogurt, 1 cup

Instruction

1. Mix all ingredients in a blender, then blend on high speed until the mixture is smooth.

2. Pour in a big, chilled glass bottle.

3. Yeast Rolls

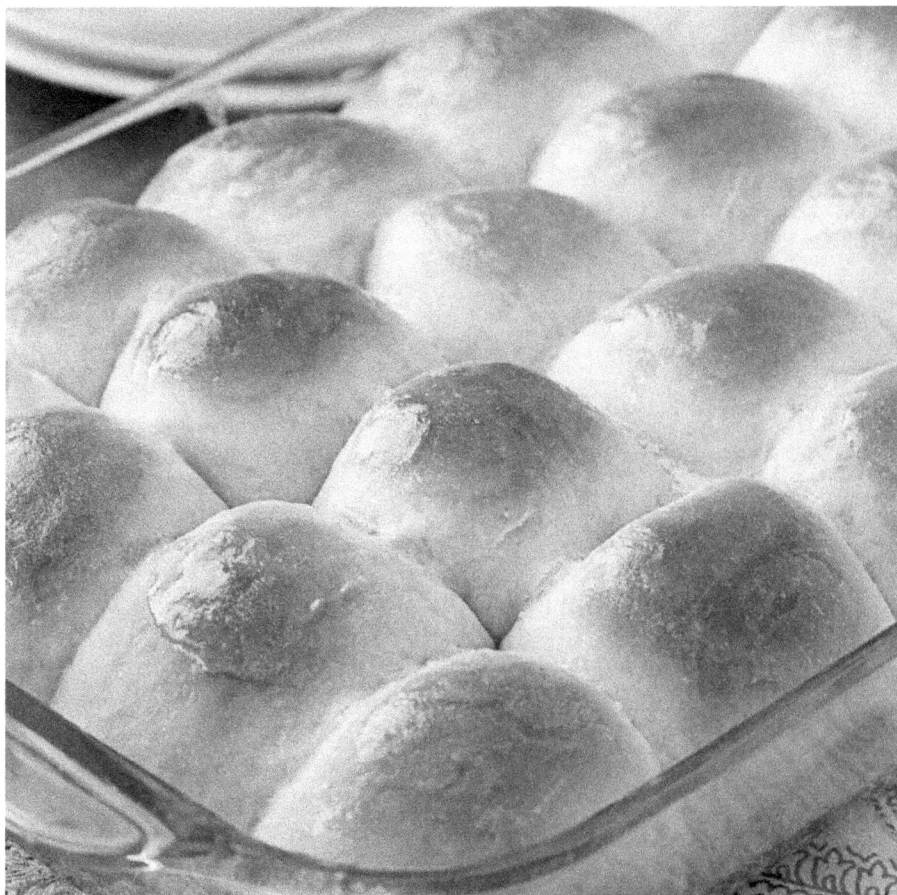

|Calories:148 | Total time: 45min | Servings: 20 | Difficulty: Easy

Ingredients

- Hot water, 1 cup

- Vegetable shortening, 6 tablespoons

- Sugar, ½ cup

- Yeast, 1 package

- Of warm water, 2 tablespoons

- 1 egg

- All-purpose flour, 3 ¾-4 cups

Instruction

1. Preheat the oven to 400 degrees F.

2. In a wide bowl, mix hot water with shortening and sugar. Put aside to cool in a safe place.

3. Dissolve the yeast in hot water.

4. Add the milk, yeast, and flour (only half of it) into the mixture, use a wide bowl and beat it well.

5. Mix the remaining flour using a spoon until it is simple to treat.

6. Place the dough in a bowl that is already greased and cover it with plastic wrap.

7. Allow to rest for 1 to 1 1/2 hours or till the dough becomes double in size.

8. Cut the sum into the required amount to shape the rolls.

9. Bake the rolls for about 12 minutes until it is completely cooked

4. Craisins with Baked Apples

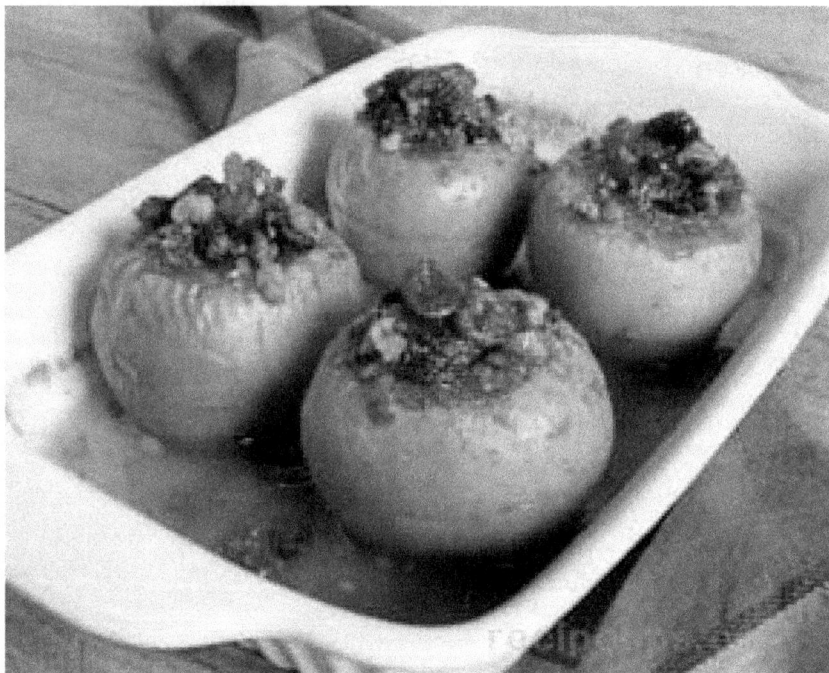

|Calories:200 | Total time: 55min | Servings: 4 | Difficulty: Easy

Ingredients

- 2 apples

- Apple juice, 1 cup

- Brown sugar packed, ¼ cup

- Craisins, 2 tablespoons

- Few red cinnamons candy

Instruction

1. Preheat to 375 Fan ovens.

2. Clean the apples and put them aside.

3. Use a square pan (size 9" x 9" x 1 3⁄4"), add apple juice with brown sugar.

4. Place the apples in the pan.

5. Cover apple centers with craisins with some cinnamon candies.

6. Now Place the pan into the microwave. Spoon sometimes adds some juice over apples for glazing during baking to stop your apples from drying.

7. Bake for around 40 to 45 minutes or till the apples is crispy when punctured with a fork.

4. Pan Sausage

|Calories:96 |Total time: 10min | Servings: 6 | Difficulty: Easy

Ingredients

- Fresh lean ground meat (beef, chicken, or turkey), 1-pound

- Ground sage, 2 teaspoons

- Granulated sugar, 2 teaspoons

- Ground black pepper, 1 teaspoon

- Ground red pepper, ½ teaspoon

- Basil (optional), 1 teaspoon

- Cooking spray

Instruction

1. Demand the butcher for meat loins of your choice.

2. Mix all the ingredients well to render the sausage.

3. Measure 2 teaspoons of the meat mixture to render a patty.

4. Pan fry or broil it until cooked properly.

5. Mexican Egg & Tortilla Skillet Breakfast (Mega)

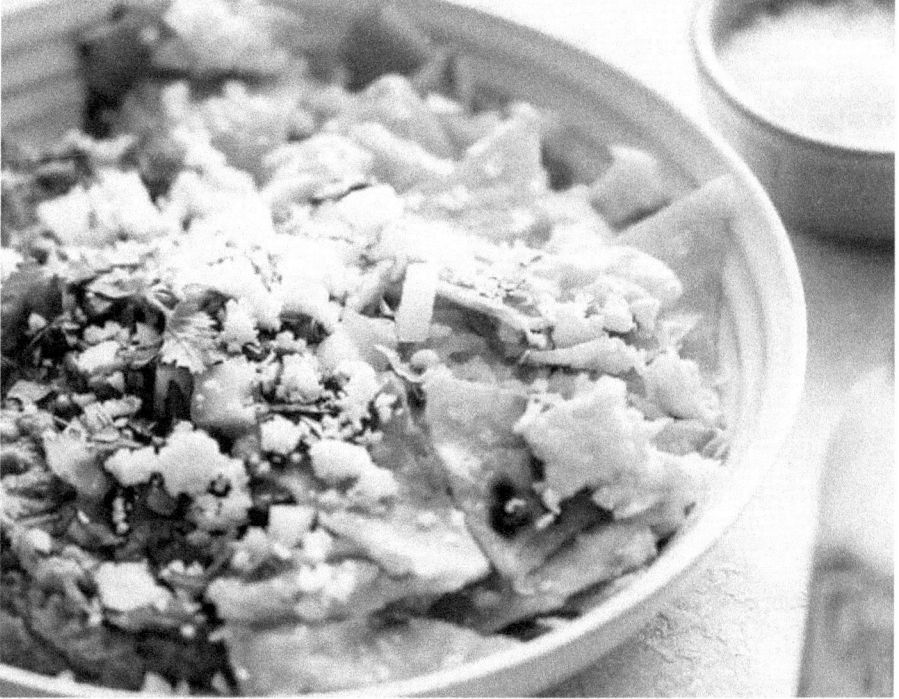

|Calories:297 | Total time: 10min | Servings:6 | Difficulty: Easy

Ingredients

- Eggs or eggbeaters, 8

- Green onions 2, make thin slices

- Chili powder, 1 teaspoon

- Low salt ketchup, 1/4 cup

- Butter, 2 tablespoons

- Unsalted tortilla chips 1 bag (6oz) *, broken up

Instruction

1. Beat the eggs until mixed.

2. Add the onion with chili powder and some ketchup. Beat again before it is well combined. Set it aside.

3. Melt some butter in a pan, then add tortilla chips and Sautee over medium heat until it is soft. Stir in the mixture of eggs and scramble till the ideal consistency is achieved. Serve hot.

* If you cannot locate unsalted tortilla chips, you may use flour tortillas and break them in fourths. Finally, Bake them until crisp at a temperature of 350°F.

6. Fresh Fruit Compote

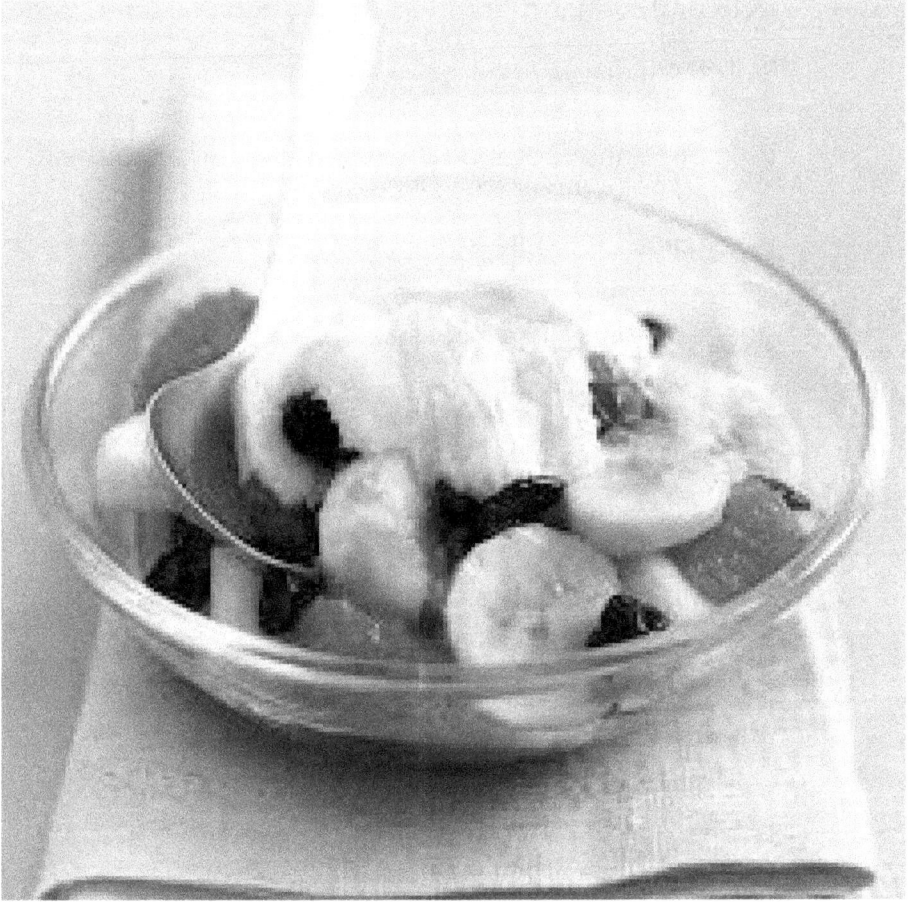

| Calories:44| Total time: 15min | Servings: 8 | Difficulty: Easy

Ingredients

- Fresh or frozen strawberries, 1/2 cup

- Fresh or frozen blackberries, 1/2 cup

- Fresh or frozen blueberries,1/2 cup

- Pared, cut peaches, 1/2 cup

- Fresh or frozen red raspberries, 1/4 cup, sweetened but not thawed

- Fresh or canned, orange juice, 1/2 cup, unsweetened

- Apple, sliced into bite-size pieces 1

- Banana, 1 sliced into bite-size pieces

Instruction

1. Add orange juice in a big container.

2. Add all the ingredients and mix gently.

3. Allow resting at room temperature for 4 hours. For thawing, use frozen berries.

7. Mexican Sausage with Eggs and Burritos

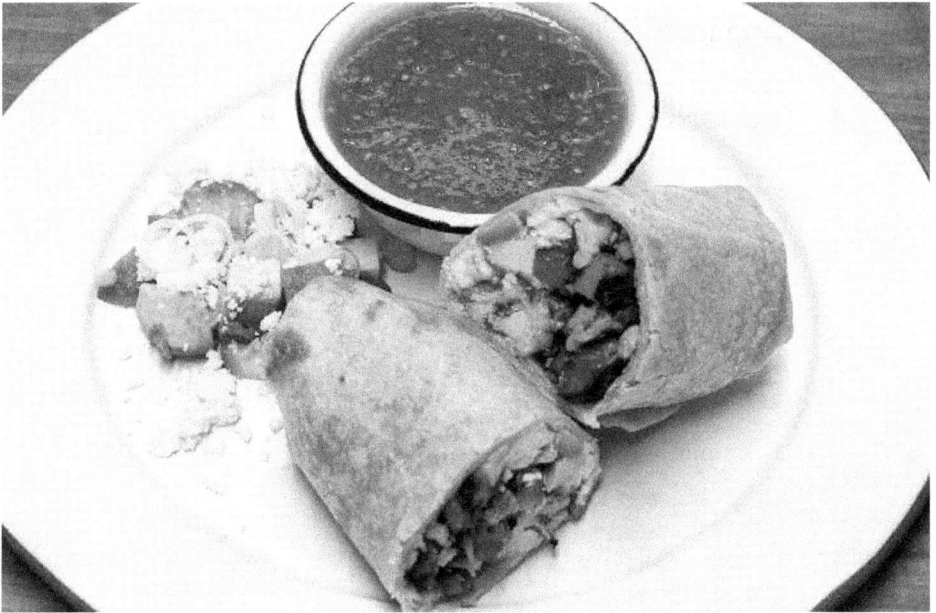

|Calories:320k| Total time: 15min | Servings: 3 | Difficulty: Easy

Ingredients

- (Mexican sausage) chorizo, 3 ounces

- Beaten eggs, 3

- Flour tortillas, 3

Instruction

1. Fry chorizo in a medium sizes skillet until the color gets dark.

2. Add the eggs and cook them until done.

3. Fill the hot tortillas using the mixture and roll them up. Now fold the bottom edge while rolling to prevent the filling from spilling out.

4. The server right away.

8. Orange Flavored Coffee

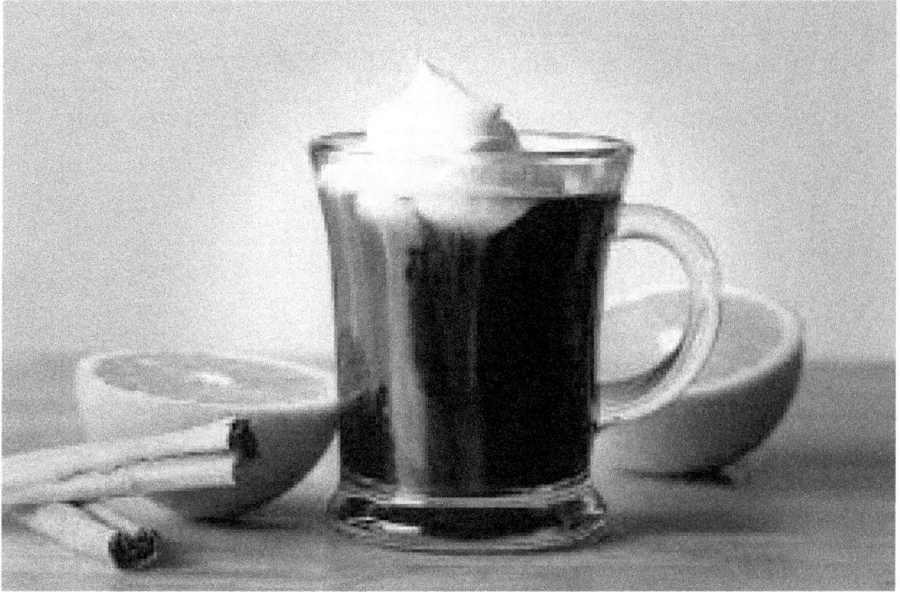

|Calories:47k | Total time: 5min | Servings: 20 | Difficulty: Easy

Ingredients

- Instant coffee, 1/2 cup

- Sugar, 3/4 cup

- Coffee-mate powder 1 cup

- Dried orange peel, 1/2 teaspoon

Instruction

1. Blend   all the   listed ingredients using   a   high-speed blender until the powdered form is achieved.

2. Place 2 circular teaspoons of the coffee mixture in a cup with each serving; finally, add the Boiling water to it

9. Caramel Rolls

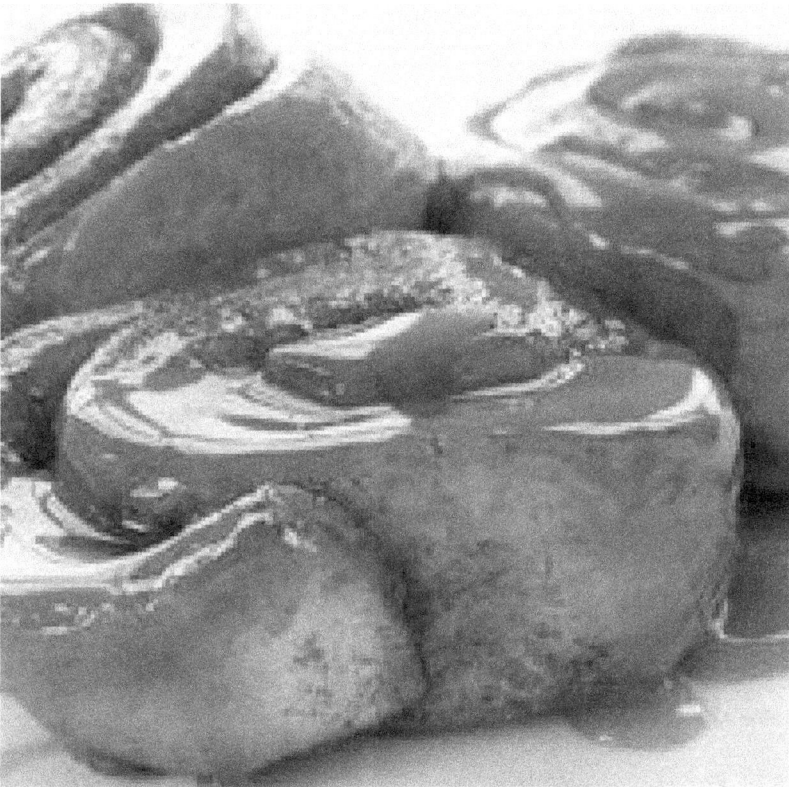

|Calories:137| Total time: 33min | Servings:24 | Difficulty: Medium-High

Ingredients

Sweet roll dough

- Flour, 2 c.

- Active dry yeast 1 pkg

- Skim milk, 1 c.

- Sugar, 1/3 c.

- Margarine, 3 Tablespoon.

- Salt, 1/4 Teaspoon

- Egg whites of 2

- Flour, 2 - 2 1/2 c.

Sauce

- Packed brown sugar, 1/2 c.

- Margarine, 3 tablespoons

- Light corn syrup 2 tablespoon

- Sugar, 1/3 c.

- Ground cinnamon, 1 teaspoon.

- Margarine melted, 1 tablespoon.

Instruction

1. Use a large bowl and add 2 cups of flour in it with yeast and set aside.

2. Mix milk, sugar, and margarine with some salt in a small size saucepan.

3. Heat and stir the mixture over low heat to melt margarine; once melted, add it to the flour blend.

4. Add whites of egg, now beat the eggs for 30 seconds with electrical beater, at medium speed, then beat for 50 seconds or more at full speed.

5. Use a spoon and add 2 – 2 1/2 cups of flour to it.

6. Knead the residual flour on a washed surface with some flour roughly spread for making a smooth dough. You will need moderately soft dough, which will be made in 3 to 5 minutes.

7. Shape the dough into a ball.

8. Spray cooking oil in a large non-stick coated bowl. Put the dough; turn it once.

9. Cover the dough with a cloth and let it rise by placing it in a warm area for about an hour; it should be twice the original size. Punch down dough with a toothpick, turn to a slightly blurred surface.

10. Split the dough into half.

11. Cover and leave 10 minutes to rest.

12. When the dough rises, mix brown sugar in a small-sized saucepan, add 3 Tablespoons. Margarine.

13. Add Maize syrup. Cook and mix the compound until the margarine is fully melted and mix. Divide dough between 2 9-inch panels

14. Spread across panes; set aside panels.

15. Use a small bowl and mix sugar with cinnamon together.

16. Roll half of the dough into a triangle measuring 12 x 8 inches.

17. Brush it with margarine previously melted; sprinkle a little bit of sugar and some cinnamon.

18. Roll up like a jelly roll look from 1 side of the rim. Pinch edges to seal together.

19. Roll cut the pieces into twelve bits. In the previously prepared panes, put cut sides down.

20. Repeat the same process with the other half leftover dough. Now Cover it with a clean dish

   towel, then allow to restore about 30 minutes.

21. Preheat the oven at 375°F pinch any bubble with a greased toothpick on the surface.

22. Bake for 20 minutes in a 375 °F oven bakes until sounding hollow when lightly tapped.

23. Invert the rolls on the platters to be served.

10. Apple Cinnamon Maple Granola

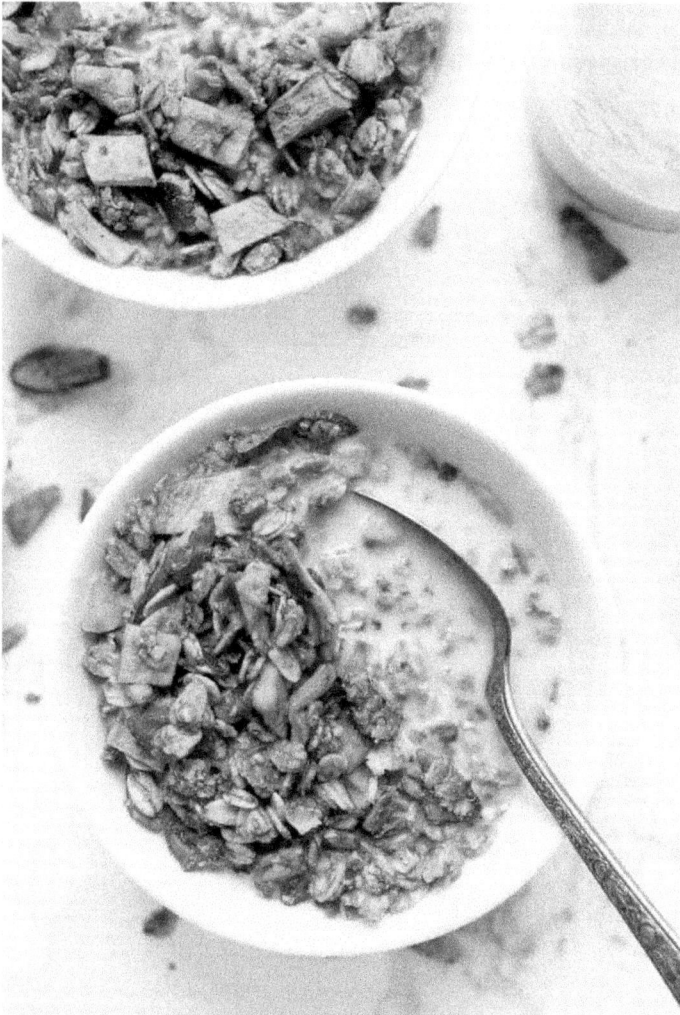

|Calories:162| Total time: 2hour | Servings:2 | Difficulty: Easy

Ingredients

- Puffed rice cereal, 3 cups

- Old fashioned oats, 3 cups

- Apple chips baked, 3.4-ounce package

- Sweetened cranberries dried, 1/2 cup

- Ground cinnamon, 1-1/2 teaspoons

- Ground nutmeg, 1 teaspoon

- Coconut oil melted, 1/4 cup

- Maple syrup pure, 1/4 cup

- Vanilla extract, 1-1/2 teaspoons

- Apple sauce unsweetened, 1/2 cup

Instruction

1. Preheat your oven around 275 F. Line 2 wide sheets of parchment paper for baking.

2. In a wide bowl, mix the dried ingredients.

3. In a small cup, combine the wet ingredients.

4. Pour the wet ingredients into a bowl of dried ingredients. To coat the dry ingredients, blend them well.

5. Using 2 baking sheets, break the mixture into half.

6. Bake for 60 to 65 minutes, adjusting the pan's position (moving the pan to the lower rack

from the top rack) halfway through the baking process.

Chapter 2: Kidney Friendly Renal Diet Lunch Recipes

1. Burritos Rapidos

|Calories:232| Total time: 10min | Servings: 4 | Difficulty: Easy

Ingredients

- Olive or canola oil, 1 1/2 teaspoons

- Diced bell pepper, red 1/2

- Thin slices of onions (scallions), green4

- Beaten eggs, 8

- Corn tortillas, (6-inch) 4

Instruction

1. Heat the oil in a medium-size frying pan over medium heat.

2. Add the bell pepper and the green onion and roast for around 3 minutes or until softened.

3. Add the eggs, then scramble for about five min or until the eggs are completely cooked.

4. Place tortillas between the two wet towel papers and place them on a tray.

5. Finally, Microwave tortillas for two minutes.

6. Spoon the egg mixture to the hot tortillas.

7. Roll up these tortillas and enjoy yourself.

8. Try applying a splash of hot sauce and sprinkle some chili powder for a slightly rich taste.

2. Buttermilk Ranch Dressing

|Calories:83g| Total time: 30min | Servings: 2 | Difficulty: Easy

Ingredients

- Mayonnaise, 1/2 cup

- Milk, 1/2 cup

- Vinegar, 2 tablespoons

- Chopped fresh chives, 1 tablespoon

- Dill, 1 tablespoon

- Chopped oregano leaves, 1 tablespoon

- Garlic powder, 1/4 teaspoon

Instruction

1. In a medium cup, whisk the mayonnaise with cream and vinegar.

2. Add fresh chips with dill, oregano leaves and 1/4 teaspoon of garlic powder.

3. Mix it.

4. Chill for at least 1 hour to encourage the flavors to mature.

5. Stir in the dressing just before eating.

3. Canned Fish Tacos

|Calories:155| Total time: 10min | Servings: 2 | Difficulty: Easy

Ingredients

- Chopped onion, 2 tablespoons

- Oil, 2 teaspoons

- Tuna rinsed, 1 can

- Canned or frozen corn, 1/2 cup

- Diced canned tomatoes, 1/4 cup without salt

- Chili powder, 1/2 teaspoon

- Corn tortillas, 4

Instruction

1. Use a frying pan and cook the onion with the oil over medium flame until onions become clear in color.

2. Add fish, maize, tomatoes, and chili powder.

3. Cook until it is heated throughout, around 3-5 minutes.

4. Serve with some soft tortillas. If needed, Add sour cream it and lettuce with hot sauce.

5. You can swap canned tuna with canned salmon. If not, then chicken may be used. You may consider using 1/2 Teaspoon of onion powder instead of fresh onion.

4. Carrot Muffins

|Calories:206 |Total time: 30min | Servings: 8 | Difficulty: Easy

Ingredients

- All-purpose flour, 1/2 cup

- Whole wheat flour, 1/2 cup

- Oats, 1/2 cup

- Ground flaxseed, 1/4 cup optional

- Baking powder, 3/4 teaspoon

- Baking soda, 3/4 teaspoon

- Cinnamon, 3/4 teaspoon

- Ginger (optional) ,1/2 teaspoon

- Brown sugar, 1/2 cup

- Vegetable oil, 1/2 cup

- Eggs, 2 larges

- Unsweetened applesauce, 1/2 cup

- Fresh ginger (optional), 2-inch piece

- Shredded carrots (~6 medium sizes) 2 cups

Instruction

1. Preheat the oven to 350 °

2. Coat the muffin tins slightly with some oil or non-stick spray.

3. Mix the dry ingredients in a large bowl.

4. Use a fork or whisk to combine the moist ingredients in a medium dish.

5. Stir the wet ingredients into the dry ingredients before they are mixed.

6. Add in shredded carrots meanwhile, stir occasionally

7. Cover the muffins with the batter evenly.

8. Bake for approximately 20 minutes.

5. Corn and Chicken Chowder

Calories:472 |Total time: 32min | Servings: 6 | Difficulty: Easy

Ingredients

- Bacon (low sodium), 12 slices

- Chopped onions, 2

- Low sodium chicken broth, 7 cups

- Diced and soaked potatoes, 4

- Corn, 8 cups

- Diced chicken breasts boneless, 8

- Fresh chopped thyme, 6 tablespoons

- Mocha mix, 4 cups

- black pepper, 1/2 teaspoon

- Green chopped onions, 8

Instruction

1. Cook the bacon in the skillet until it is crisply cut the bacon and put aside.

2. Sautee the slices of onions in the fat of the bacon

3. Add the butter and the potatoes.

4. Cover and cook for 10 minutes.

5. Add some maize, chicken, and thyme.

6. Now Cover and boil till the chicken is cooked; it will take around 15 minutes.

7. Mix in the broth and boil for 2 minutes.

8. Sprinkle with sausage, pepper, and some green onions.

6. Chicken and Dumplings

|Calories:401|Total time: 8hour | Servings: 6 | Difficulty: Easy

Ingredients

- Whole chicken, 1 or chopped chicken, 3 lbs.

- Chicken broth or, 2 cups of water

- Finely cut celery leaves, 1 stalk

- Sliced carrots, 2-3

- Black pepper, 1/2 teaspoon

- Mace or nutmeg, 1/2 teaspoon

- 1/4 cup flour

- Eggs, 2

- Milk, 2/3 cup

- Baking powder, 3 teaspoons

- Flour, 2 cups

- Margarine or unsalted butter, 2 tablespoons

Instruction

1. Put chicken and vegetables with some spices, then add water or chicken broth in a cooker.

2. Add more water, sufficient to cover the chicken with around 1".

3. Put the cooker on slow heat for around 6-8 hours.

4. Put the chicken in the ovenproof bowl.

5. If you like, then remove the bones, or they may just fall off automatically.

6. Cover and keep it warm.

7. Turn the cooker heat to high. Now add 1/4 cup of flour and whisk rapidly to prevent lumps.

8. Break the butter into 2 cups with a knife.

9. Mix the wet ingredients for a stiff dough and add a spoon of boiling broth.

10. Cover the pot, reduce the heat to stop boiling, now cook slowly for 15 mins without removing the cap.

11. Place chicken inside a large serving dish then pours over the thickened sauce. Serve with dumplings.

7. Chicken Lasagna and White Sauce

|Calories:453| Total time: 60min | Servings: 6 | Difficulty: Easy

Ingredients

- Chicken breast or thigh, 6 oz.

- Chicken broth 12 ounces low sodium

- Olive oil, 1/4 cup

- Diced onion, 1 large

- Oregano, 1 tablespoon

- Black pepper, 1/4 teaspoon

- White wine (optional), 1/4 cup

- Thick-sliced mushrooms, 1/2 cup

- Flour, 3 tablespoons

- Cream cheese, 6 ounces

- Mocha mix, 1 1/2 cups

- Nutmeg, 1/4-1/2 teaspoon

- Fresh parmesan cheese, grated 1/2 cup

- Sliced into little moons, 1 1/2 zucchini,

- Lasagna noodles not boiled, 1 package

Instruction

1. Preheat oven to 325 F.

2. Put chicken and stock in a small pan, then bring to a boil, now reduce heat and simmer once chicken becomes white and thoroughly cooked. The chicken cooks

   better if it is sliced into bits.

3. In the meantime, add some olive oil, oregano with onions, then add black pepper in a wide saucepan over medium heat, Now sauté everything for 5 min or until the onion starts to soften.

4. Add to the pan some wine and encourage to evaporate it.

5. Add the mushrooms.

6. Sprinkle the flour evenly over the plate, mixing slightly to scatter the flavors.

7. Now on low heat, cook about 3 minutes

8. Split the cream cheese and return it to the pan, stirring it again until it is melted and uniformly spread. (~2 min.)

9. Slowly add the Mocha mixture to the plate, stirring again.

10. Ingredients should now be thickening, not clumpy. If it is all clumpy, carry on stirring to split them up.

11. Add some nutmeg.

12. Stir in now parmesan cheese and keep stirring while it heats for another 5 mins. The sauce must also be thickened.

13. Take the chicken out from the pot (save the broth), use two knives, break the chicken and attempt to hold the bits intact.

14. Put it aside. Stir in half a cup of the remaining broth into the cream mixture while stirring regularly for 2 minutes.

15. Put the lasagna sheets on the pan, cover with 1/3 sauce, add 1/2 of the chicken with 1/2 of the parts of the zucchini, spread thinly on top.

16. Cover with foil, put it in the oven for around 30 minutes and cut the foil before crisp.

8. Chicken Seafood Gumbo

|Calories:240|Total time: 45min | Servings:6 | Difficulty: Easy

Ingredients

- Canola oil, 1 tablespoon

- Chopped celery stalks, 3

- Chopped yellow onion, 1

- Chopped bell pepper red, 1

- Chopped chicken breasts skinless, 2

- Sliced lean smoked turkey sausage 8 ounces,

- Canola oil, 1/2 cup

- Flour, 1/2 cup

- Cajun seasoning salt-free, 1 tablespoon

- Chicken broth low sodium 2 quarts

- Cooked shrimp, 1/2 pound

- Canned crab, 6 ounces

- Chopped frozen okra, 3 cups

Instruction

1. Heat about 1 tablespoon of canola oil in 4.5-quarter or a larger pot over medium heat.

2. Add the celery, cabbage, clove pepper with chicken and sausage and simmer for about 10 minutes.

3. Take the mixture out of the pot and put it aside.

4. Decrease the heat to medium.

5. Now add about 1/2 cup of canola oil, then add some flour to make the roux.

6. Stir in the Cajun seasoning and simmer for 1 minute or more it depends on how much dark you like.

7. Slowly mix in chicken broth while constantly stirring to prevent lumps.

8. Increase the heat to medium level and allow the mixture to boil for around 10 minutes or before it begins to thicken slightly.

9. Reduce heat now to medium and then add crabs, okra, and chicken mixture back to the pot.

10. Cook for about 10 minutes or until the mixture is properly heated

9. Cornbread Stuffing with Chicken

|Calories:372| Total time: 1.5hour | Servings: 4 | Difficulty: Easy

Ingredients

- Fresh parsley, 1 tablespoon

- 2 tablespoons, Dash (original blend) + 1 1/2 teaspoons extra

- Mrs. Dash (chicken grilling blend), 1 tablespoon

- Skinless boneless, chicken breast, 4 (4 ounces) pieces

- Unsalted butter, 1 tablespoon

- Chopped celery, 1 cup

- Chopped onion, 1/2 cup

- Ground sage, 2 teaspoons

- Coarsely crumbled cornbread, 2 cups (about 7 ounces)

- Unseasoned croutons, 2 cups

- chicken broth (low sodium), 1 cup

Instruction

1. Chop the parsley.

2. Mix 1 tablespoon of Mrs. Dash® (Original Blend) with Mrs. Dash® (Chicken Grilling Blend) and parsley.

3. Cover chicken breasts from all sides with a blend of seasoning.

4. Spray on a large non-stick stove some cooking spray.

5. Heat the skillet over medium flame until it is hot.

6. Add the chicken breasts to the skillet, cook for 3 to 5 min each side or until lightly golden.

7. Take the chicken breasts from the skillet and put them aside.

8. Preheat the oven to 35F.

9. Melt the butter in a saucepan over low heat. Add the celery, the cabbage, 1 tablespoon + 1 1/2 Teaspoon of Mrs. Dash® (Original Blend), the sage, and the combination.

10. Cook over medium heat for 6-7 minutes or until all vegetables are soft.

11. Remove from the heat.

12. In a mixing dish, combine the cornbread crumbs and croutons.

13. Add the mixture of vegetables and the broth by swirling to combine.

14. Spoon the dressing mixture on a large baking dish lightly coated with some non-stick cooking oil.

15. Organize chicken breasts with dressing mixture.

16. Cover and bake at 350 ° for 45 minutes.

17. Remove cover and continue cooking for 5 minutes or till the chicken breast's internal temperature is around 170 degrees.

18. Garnish using leaves of celery, if needed.

Chapter 3: Kidney Friendly Renal Diet Dinner Recipes

1. Cilantro Slaw & Black Bean Burger

|Calories:380cal |Total time: 1hour| Servings: 6| Difficulty: Easy

Ingredients

- black beans, ½ cup rinsed

- Bulgur wheat, ½ cup

- Ground black pepper, 1 teaspoon

- Granulated garlic, 1 teaspoon

- Smoked paprika, ½ teaspoon

- French's® Worcestershire sauce 1 tablespoon,

- Onion flakes, 1 teaspoon

- Better than bouillon® beef, 1 tablespoon

- Onions, ½ cup

- Scallions, ¼ cup

- Flour, 2 tablespoons

- Slaw mix 3 cups (10-ounce bag) (also known as power blend)

- Balsamic vinegar, ¼ cup

- Cilantro, 2 tablespoons

- Sesame oil, 2 tablespoons

- Oil for searing*2 tablespoons canola

- Lime juice ¼ cup

- zest of, 1 lime

- Mayonnaise, ¼ cup

- Hamburger rolls, 6

Instruction

1. Preheat the oven to around 400 degrees F.

2. Mix black beans with bulgur wheat, add ground black pepper, mix it with spoon, add granulated garlic, some smoked paprika, and then add Worcestershire sauce and onion flakes 1 Teaspoon. Of water, then add beef bouillon and onions; finally, add 1⁄2 cup of scallions in a medium-sized dish.

3. Melt around 1⁄2 cup of the mixture in the burgers and refrigerate it until solid (not frozen).

4. Create vinaigrette with a combination of vinegar, add one tablespoon of cilantro with sesame oil and the lime juice.

5. Add 2 teaspoons of vinaigrette into the slaw mixture in a small pot, blend gently, and put aside in the refrigerator.

6. In another little bowl, combine the mayonnaise with the vinaigrette's remaining 2 teaspoons and put it aside.

7. Dust the black bean burgers using some flour and extract any waste. Bake for about 14 minutes and turn burgers halfway round.

8. Toast the rolls and scatter the same volume of the can. Add black bean burgers and finish with around 1⁄4 cup (or desired quantity) of slaw.

2. Smoky Cheese Sauce with Shrimp Grit Cakes & Egg

|Calories:390cal |Total time: 1.5hour| Servings:6 | Difficulty: Easy

Ingredients

- Beaten eggs, 4

- Unsalted butter, 2 tablespoons

- Diced onions, ½ cup

- Bacon½-inch pieces, 4 slices

- Deveined and peeled shrimp 12 16/20 count,

- Old bay® seasoning ,1 teaspoon

- Chopped chives, ¼ cup

- Chicken stock without salt, ½ cup,

- "better than bouillon" ® 2 teaspoons chicken flavor,

- 1 cup milk

- Grits, ½ cup

- Canola oil, 2 tablespoons

- Ground black pepper, ½ teaspoon

- Smoked paprika, ½ teaspoon

- Shredded cheddar cheese, ¼ cup

- Havarti, ¼ cup

- Canola oil, ¼ cup

- Flour, 3 tablespoons

Instruction

1. Heat the canola oil in a broad non-stick sauté pan, then scramble the eggs until cooked, not be too dry.

2. Place aside in the medium dish. Add the butter to the pan, then sauté the onions with shrimp, Old Bay®, then simply add about half of the chips until shrimps are slightly yellow.

3. Add chicken broth, eggs, and grits with bouillon and cook until finished according to box

   instructions.

4. Turn off the heat and fold the egg, the bacon, and the shrimp mixture in the bowl. Place the mixture in lightly oiled baking dish 9" x 9" size and spread it until even

coating is achieved, then cover and refrigerate it until solid.

5. Take the pan and break it into 6 squares.

6. Use a saucepan and heat the milk until it becomes hot. Now whisk in the cheese, the ground black pepper, some paprika and all the remaining chips until melted.

7. Place the sauce aside.

8. Heat half of the canola oil in a wide saucepan.

9. Lightly dust the grated cakes with flour and sauté them until they get golden brown.

10. Plate with equivalent quantities of smoked cheese sauce at the end

3. Bavarian Pot Roast Slow-Cooked

|Calories:313cal |Total time: 8.5hour| Servings: 12| Difficulty: Medium

Ingredients

- Beef chuck roast, 3 pounds

- Vegetable oil, 1 teaspoon

- Fresh ground ginger, ½ teaspoon

- Pepper, ½ teaspoon

- Whole cloves, 3

- Sliced apples, 2 cups

- Sliced onions, ½ cup

- Apple juice, ½ cup

- Flour, 4 tablespoons

- Water, 4 tablespoons

- Fresh apple slices for garnish

Instruction

1. Strip the beef roast from the extra fat.

2. Rinse and drain the pat. Rub some oil over the roast's top, now brush with ginger & pepper, then add the entire cloves.

3. Caramelize the pot roast using a hot oil pan on both sides.

4. Put the apples and the onions in a crock-pot.

5. Add the pot roast to and spill the apple juice all over the whole roast.

6. Cover and cook at low heat for 2 hours or maybe more depending upon the situation

7. Remove the roast from the slow cooker. Put it away but hold it warm. Strain the casserole juices and place them into the slow cooker again.

8. Switch the heat up to medium and thicken the liquid.

9. Create a smooth paste using flour and water, add to cooker.

10. Cover and boil until the mixture is thickened. Just before dinner, spill over the roast.

4. Spicy Beef Stir-Fry

|Calories:261cal |Total time: 25min| Servings: 4| Difficulty: Easy

Ingredients

- Separated cornstarch, 2 Tablespoons

- Sesame oil, ¼ teaspoon

- Sugar, ½ teaspoon

- Water, 2 tablespoons

- Large egg, 1

- Canola oil, 3 tablespoons

- Sliced beef round tip, 12 ounces

- Sliced green bell pepper, 1

- Sliced onions, 1 cup

- Ground chili pepper red, ¼ teaspoon

- Sherry, 1 tablespoon

- Soy sauce, 2 teaspoons

- Parsley as per need

Instruction

1. In a big bowl, whisk about 1 tablespoon of cornstarch, 1 & half tablespoon of water, 1 large egg size, 1 tablespoon of canola oil, and the beef. Now marinate for about 20 minutes.

2. In a separate cup, mix the leftover cornstarch with the water. Set it aside.

3. Heat 2 teaspoons of canola oil and add all the mixture to it (use a small saucepan for this). Cook it until the meat starts to brown.

4. Add orange bell pepper and the onion with some chili pepper. Finally, add the sherry. Cook about one minute. Add soya sauce, sugar, and some sesame oil.

5. Zesty Orange Tilapia

|Calories:133cal |Total time: 25min | Servings: 4 | Difficulty: Easy

Ingredients

- Tilapia, 16 ounces

- Julienned carrots, 1 cup

- Julienned celery, ¾ cup

- Sliced green onions, ½ cup

- Grated orange peel, 2 teaspoons

- Orange juice, 4 teaspoons

- Ground black pepper, 1 teaspoon

Instruction

1. Preheat the oven to 450 degrees F.

2. Mix broccoli, green onions with celery, and zest of the orange in a small bowl.

3. Break the tilapia into four equal parts.

4. Tear off four-wide squares of a foil and coat the foil with non-stick spray.

5. On each sheet of foil, put 1⁄4 of vegetables slightly off the middle and then top with the fish.

6. Now Sprinkle 1 Teaspoon of orange juice over each top. Season with some black pepper.

7. Fold the foil around the sides to create an envelope and put the foil right on the baking sheet.

8. Bake for around 10 minutes. When finished, fish can split quickly with a fork.

9. Remove the bags and put them directly on plates.

10. Be alert when you open because of the steam.

6. Mashed Carrots with Ginger

|Calories:30cal | Total time: 15min | Servings: 3| Difficulty: Easy

Ingredients

- Baby carrots, 2 cups

- Chopped fresh ginger, ½ teaspoon

- Honey, ½ teaspoon

- Black pepper, ½ teaspoon

- Vanilla extract, ½ teaspoon

- Optional for garnish: fresh chives, 1 tablespoon.

Instruction

1. Boil or steam the carrots at high flame until the carrots are soft.

2. Drop heat to medium and mash all the carrots with the masher.

3. Add the remaining ingredients, i.e. (honey, ginger, vanilla extract with pepper), then mix until well combined.

7. Aromatic Herbed Rice

|Calories: 134cal |Total time: 5min| Servings:6| Difficulty: Easy

Ingredients

- Olive oil, 2 tablespoons

- Rice 3 cups, cooked (do not overcook)

- Garlic 4–5 cloves, fresh and sliced thin

- Cilantro 2 tablespoons, fresh and sliced

- Oregano 2 tablespoons, fresh and sliced

- Chives 2 tablespoons, fresh and sliced

- Red pepper flakes, ½ teaspoon

- Red wine vinegar, 1 teaspoon

Instruction

1. In a wide saucepan, heat the olive oil over a medium-high flame and sauté the garlic gently. Add now rice, herbs, and red pepper flakes, then simmer for about 2–4 minutes or until well blended.

2. Turn the heat off, add the vinegar, blend well and serve.

3. Chicken and Dumplings

8. Easy chicken on a slow cooker

|Calories:401cal |Total time:20min | Servings:6 | Difficulty: Easy

Ingredients

- Chicken 1 whole or chicken 3 lbs., sliced

- Water 2 cups of chicken broth low sodium

- Celery with leaves 1 stalk, cut fine

- Carrots 2-3, sliced

- Black pepper, 1/2 teaspoon

- Mace or nutmeg, 1/2 teaspoon

- Flour, 1/4 cup

- Eggs, 2

- Milk, 2/3 cup

- Baking powder, 3 teaspoons

- Flour, 2 cups

- Butter or margarine, 2 tablespoons, unsalted

Instruction

1. Take a slow cooker, then put the chicken, the vegetables, spices, and water inside it.

2. Add more water, sufficient to cover the chicken with around 1.

3. Switch the cooker on low flame for around 6-8 hours.

4. Take the chicken out from the ovenproof bowl.

5. Remove bones from meat. If you like, they may just slip off.

6. Cover and hold it wet.

7. Turn the slow cooker to increased heat. Add 1/4 cup of flour and whisk rapidly to prevent lumps.

8. Slice the butter with a knife and put it in two cups of flour.

9. Mix in wet ingredients for a firm dough and add the spoonful of it to the boiling broth.

10. Cover the cooker, lower the heat to stop boiling, then cook for about 15 minutes without uncovering it.

11. Place chicken in a wide serving plate and pour over the thickened sauce. Now serve it with dumplings.

9. Kidney Friendly Vegetable Soup

|Calories: 42Kcal |Total time: 50min| Servings:5| Difficulty: Easy

Ingredients

- Onion 1 medium, (150g / 6oz)

- Carrots 6 large, (6 x 140g / 5 ½ oz)

- Turnip 1 medium, (110g / 4 ½ oz)

- Celery 2 sticks, (60g / 2oz)

- Garlic 2 large cloves

- Chicken or vegetable low stock dices 1, a very little salt

- Bay leaf, 1

- Thyme, 1 teaspoon, fresh and sliced

- Black pepper, ¼ teaspoon

- Olive oil, 1 tablespoon

- Water 1 – 1.2 L

Instruction

1. Peel the onion, the carrot, and the turnip, then finely chop (for this, a food processor can accelerate the chopping process)

2. Dice the garlic and the celery finely.

3. Put the thinly sliced carrot, turnip inside a big pot, and then add water of about 4 times of their volume. Bring it to boil and cook until tender.

4. During when carrot and the turnip are frying, flame the olive oil in the frying pan.

5. Now add the onion, garlic, and celery once the oil is quietly hot. Put the vegetables in oil with a spoon to coat them.

6. Cover the pan with the lid and leave for half-fry over a low flame until softened. It is going to take around 15 minutes.

7. Shake or open the pot from about time to time, then mix to make sure it is burning or stuck.

8. Add the boiling carrot with turnip and blend.

9. Making chicken or vegetable stock via adding one very low salted vegetable or as per choice chicken stock cube into 1-1,2 Liter of boiling water.

10. Put the stock in the mixture of vegetables

11. Add now the bay leaf to the thyme

12. Season with some pepper

13. Put to a boil, after this cook for thirty min (or until the vegetables are cooked) without covering with a lid.

14. Drop the leaf of the Bay. Mix the broth until creamy by using a food processor.

15. Extra water may be applied to getting a thin soup.

Chapter 4: Kidney Friendly Renal Diet Dessert Recipes

1. Strawberry Sorbet

Calories: 22 kcal| Total time: 4 hr.| Serving: 3| Difficulty: Easy

Ingredients

- Date Sugar, ½ cup

- Strawberries, 2 cups

- Spring Water, 2 cups

- Spelt Flour, 1 ½ teaspoon.

Instructions

1. Begin by combing date sugar, spelled flour, and spring water in a medium-sized pot. Next, heat the mixture over low heat and cook for 8 to 10 minutes or till thickened. After that, take off the pot from the heat and allow it to cool. Once cooled, puree the strawberries in a blender.

2. Now, mix the strawberry puree to the flour mixture and give everything a good stir. Then, pour the mixture into a container and keep it in the freezer. Cut the frozen sorbet to pieces and place it in the blender or food processor.

3. Blend until smooth and return the container to the refrigerator for a minimum of 4 hours.

4. Finally, serve the chilled strawberry sorbet.

2. Strawberry Ice Cream

Calories: 354 kcal| Total time: 20 mins| Serving: 3-4| Difficulty: Medium

Ingredients

- Hemp Milk, ¼ cup

- Frozen strawberries, 1 cup

- Agave Syrup, 1 tablespoon.

- Frozen Baby, Bananas, 5

- Ripe Avocado, ½ of 1

Instructions

1. Place all ingredients necessary to make this ice cream into a high-speed blender. Mix them for 2-3 minutes or till the mixture is smooth.

2. Check for sugar and, if appropriate, insert more agave syrup.

3. Finally, move to the freezer-friendly jar and freeze for 4-6 hours

3. Blueberry Muffins

Calories: 383 kcal| Total time: 14 mins| Serving: 12| Difficulty: Easy

Ingredients

- Two and a half cup, almond flour

- One-third cup, keto-friendly sugar

- One and a half teaspoon, baking powder

- Half teaspoon, baking soda

- Half teaspoon, kosher salt

- One-third cup, melted butter

- One-third cup, unsweetened almond milk

- Three large eggs

- One teaspoon, pure vanilla extract

- Two-third cup, blueberries

- Half lemon zests

Instructions

1. Start by preheating the oven to a temperature of 350 ° and put in a muffin tray with cupcake liners.

2. In a big container, stir together almond flour, Swerve, baking soda, baking powder, and salt. Gently stir in melted butter, eggs, and vanilla once mixed.

3. Gently fold the blueberries and the lemon zest until uniformly spread. Scoop equivalent quantities of the mixture into each liner of cupcakes and bake until softly golden. A toothpick inserted into the middle of the muffin comes out clean; this will happen within 23 minutes. Let it cool slightly before serving.

4. Gingersnap Baked Apples

Calories: 343 kcal| Total time: 1 hr.| Serving: 8| Difficulty: Easy

Ingredients

- Gingersnap cookies, 3 ounces

- Brown sugar, 2 tablespoons

- Apples, 4 sweet

- Butter rinsed, ¼ cup

- Whipping cream, ½ cup

Instructions

1. Gingersnaps and brown sugar whirl into small crumbs in the mixer or the food processor.

2. Cut around cores up to around 3/4 of the way through apples with a thin, sharp knife, beginning from stem ends; pick out cores with the spoon, creating a 1 1/2-inch-wide cavity and then keeping bases unaffected. - In the shallow 2 3-quart baking dish, set the apples moderately apart.

3. Spoon each cavity with 1 tablespoon of ginger snap mixture and finish with 1/2 tablespoon of butter. Sprinkle

the apples generously with the remaining blend of ginger.

4. Bake in a standard or convection oven of 375o until apples are soft, around 45 minutes until pierced. Shift into individual bowls and, if necessary, pour 2 teaspoons of cream around each.

5. Apple cider donut bites

Calories: 164 kcal| Time: 30 mins| Serving 12 | Difficulty: easy

Ingredients

Donut bites:

- Almond flour, 2 cups

- Swerve sweetener, ½ cup

- Whey protein powder unflavored, ¼ cup

- Baking powder, 2 teaspoons

- Cinnamon, ½ teaspoon

- Salt, ½ teaspoon

- Large eggs, 2

- Cup water, 1/3

- Butter melted, ¼ cup.

- Apple cider vinegar, 1 ½ tablespoon

- Apple extract, 1 ½ teaspoon

Coating:

- Swerve sweetener, 1/4 cup

- Cinnamon, 1 to 2 teaspoons

- Butter melted, 1/4 cup.

Instructions

1. Oven Preheated to325f, then grease well a tiny muffin pan (use a standard muffin box with 24 cavities).

2. Mix all the almond meal, sweetener, powder of protein, dried powder, spices & salt in the large bowl. Whisk till it is mixed in milk, sugar, butter, cider vinegar & apple extract.

3. Divide the mixture between the wells of the prepared tiny muffin pan. Bake for 15-20 mins, till the cup's cakes, are hard to touch. Remove & allow it to cool for 10 mins, then Switch to the wire rack to completely cool.

4. Mix both sweetener & spices in a tiny bowl. Dip a full bite of donut in the softened butter, fully covering it. Then roll the combination into each donut snap.

6. Gingersnap Baked Apples

Calories: 346 kcal| Preparation time: 1 hr.| Servings: 8 | Difficulty: Easy

Ingredients

- Gingersnap cookies, 3 ounces

- Brown sugar, 2 tablespoons

- Apples, 4 sweet

- Butter rinsed, 1/4 cup

- Whipping cream, 1/2 cup

Instructions

1. Gingersnaps and brown sugar whirl into small crumbs in the mixer or the food processor.

2. Cut around cores up to around 3/4 of the way through apples with a thin, sharp knife, beginning from stem ends; pick out cores with the spoon, creating a 1 1/2-inch-wide cavity and then keeping bases unaffected. - In the shallow 2 3-quart baking dish, set the apples moderately apart.

3. Spoon each cavity with 1 tablespoon of ginger snap mixture and finish with 1/2 tablespoon of butter. Sprinkle the apples generously with the remaining blend of ginger.

4. Bake in a standard or convection oven of 375o until apples are soft, around 45 minutes until pierced. Shift into individual bowls and, if necessary, pour 2 teaspoons of cream around each.

Chapter 5: Kidney Friendly Renal Diet Beverages

1. Strawberry Banana Smoothie

Calories: 85 kcal| Total Time: 10 minutes | Serving: 2| Difficulty: Easy

Ingredients:

1. Hemp Milk, 2 cups

2. 4 Banana

3. Dates, ¾ cup

4. Agave, 1 tablespoon.

5. Strawberry, 8 oz.

Instructions:

1. Mix the strawberries and other ingredients in a blender till they are slightly broken down.

2. Then add banana and hemp milk. Put agave. Blend till well mixed.

3. Serve and enjoy it!

2. Apple-Cinnamon Flavored Water

Calories: 4 kcal| Total Time: 12 hrs. | Serving: 8 | Difficulty: Easy

Ingredients

1. Water, 10 cups

2. Apple, 1 medium

3. Sticks, 2 cinnamon

4. Ground cinnamon, 2 teaspoons

Instructions

1. Cut a peeled apple into slices and soak all ingredients in water

2. Refrigerate overnight.

3. Serve

3. Beet and Apple Juice Blend

Calories: 53 kcal| Total Time: 5 minutes | Serving: 2 | Difficulty: Easy

Ingredients

- Apple, 1/2 medium

- Beet, 1/2 medium

- fresh carrot, 1 medium

- stalk, 1 celery

- parsley, 1/4 cup

Instructions

1. Put all ingredients in a juicer and extract the juice.

2. Transfer to a glass.

3. Enjoy!

4. Blackberry-Sage Flavored Water

Calories: 7 kcal| Total Time: 12 hrs. | Serving: 8 | Difficulty: Easy

Ingredients

- Fresh blackberries, 1 cup

- Sage leaves, 4

- Water, 10 cups

Instructions

1. Mash blackberries and add all ingredients to a pitcher.

2. Refrigerator overnight.

3. Serve and enjoy.

5. Blueberry Blast Smoothie

Calories: 108 kcal| Total Time: minutes | Serving: | Difficulty: Easy

Ingredients

- Frozen blueberries, 1 cup

- Splenda® ,8 packets

- Protein powder, 6 tablespoons

- Ice cubes ,8

- Apple juice, 14 ounces

Instructions

1. Mix all of the mentioned ingredients and blend till well-combined.

2. Serve in a glass.

6. Café au Lait Protein Wake-Up

Calories: 100 kcal| Total Time: 5 minutes | Serving: 1| Difficulty: Easy

Ingredients

1. Protein powder, 1 scoop

2. Hot coffee ,8 ounces

3. Flavored liquid ,2 tablespoons coffee creamer

Instructions

1. Place one scoop of protein powder in a cup. Add coffee and stir until dissolved.

2. Now add coffee creamer.

3. Serve and enjoy.

7. Caramel Protein Latte

Calories: 72 kcal| Total Time: 5 minutes | Serving: 1 | Difficulty: Easy

Ingredients

- Whey protein powder, 1 scoop

- Water, 2 ounces

- Hot coffee, 6 ounces

- Caramel syrup Sugar-Free, 2 tablespoons

Instructions

1. Transfer protein powder in a jug, add water and mix till dissolved.

2. Now add hot coffee and stir.

3. Now add caramel syrup.

4. Serve in a cup and enjoy.

8. Kidney friendly Chocolate Smoothie

Calories: 215 kcal| Total Time: minutes | Serving: | Difficulty: Easy

Ingredients

- Powered Bakers Cocoa, 1 tablespoon unsweetened

- Cold water, 1 tablespoon

- Sugar, 1 tablespoon

- Egg white, 8 ounces

- Whipped topping, 4 tablespoons

- Chocolate bar shavings

Instructions

1. Mix cocoa, sugar, and water. Add and mix egg whites and whipping cream till combined.

2. Serve

Chapter 6: Kidney Friendly Renal Diet Salads

1. Lemon Orzo Spring Salad

Calories: 330 kcal| Total time: 40 minutes| Servings: 4|Difficulty: Easy

Ingredients

- Orzo pasta, ¾ cup

- Fresh yellow peppers, ¼ cup, diced

- Fresh red peppers, ¼ cup, diced

- Fresh green peppers, ¼ cup, diced

- Fresh red onion, ½ cup, diced

- Fresh zucchini, 2 cups, medium-cubed

- Olive oil, ¼ cup

- Fresh lemon juice, 3 tablespoons

- Lemon zest, 1 teaspoon

- Grated parmesan cheese, 3 tablespoons

- Fresh rosemary, 2 tablespoons, chopped

- Black pepper, ½ teaspoon

- Dried oregano, ½ teaspoon

- Red pepper flakes, ½ teaspoon

Instructions

- Cook orzo pasta as directed on the box and drain.

- On medium-high heat, sauté peppers, zucchini, and onions with oil in a pan until translucent.

- Now mix lemon juice, cheese, rosemary, lemon zest, olive oil, pepper, oregano, red pepper in a bowl.

- Add vegetables and pasta into the bowl and fold it until well combined.

- Chill and serve.

2. Shrimp and Veggie Noodle Salad

Calories: 254 kcal| Total time: 50 minutes| Servings: 10|Difficulty: Medium

Ingredients

- Dry Spaghetti, 1-pound package, cooked

- Cooked cocktail shrimp, 4 cups

- Fresh scallions, sliced, 1 cup

- Fresh broccoli florets, 2 cups

- Fresh carrots, shredded, 1 cup

- Shitake mushrooms, chopped, 2 cups

- Sesame oil, 2 tablespoons

- Chili oil, 2 teaspoons

- Rice wine vinegar, ½ cup

- Fresh garlic, chopped, 2 tablespoons

- Fresh ginger, chopped, 1 tablespoon

- Soy sauce, low sodium, ¼ cup

- Lime juice, ¼ cup

Instructions

1. Transfer 1 cup soy sauce substitute in a saucepan.

2. Mix the first six ingredients in a bowl; set aside.

3. Blend other ingredients in the blender for about 1 minute.

4. Now pour dressing mixture on pasta mixture. Mix to coat well.

5. Serve

3. Crunchy Quinoa salad

Calories: 158 kcal| Total time: 40 minutes| Servings: 8|Difficulty: Easy

Ingredients

- Quinoa, 1 cup, rinsed

- Water, 2 cups

- Cherry tomatoes, diced, 5

- Cucumbers, ½ cup, seeded and diced

- Onions, chopped, 3 green

- Fresh mint, chopped, ¼ cup

- Parsley, chopped, ½ cup

- Fresh lemon juice, 2 tablespoons

- Grated lemon rind, 1 tablespoon

- Olive oil, 4 tablespoons

- Parmesan cheese, grated, ¼ cup

- Lettuce, ½ head

Instructions

1. Toast quinoa in pan on medium-high heat, stirring frequently. Add water and boil. Reduce heat and cover the pan, and simmer. Cool it.

2. Combine all remaining ingredients in a bowl. Add the cooled quinoa to the mixture.

3. Spoon mixture in the lettuce cups and sprinkle parmesan on top.

4. Serve and enjoy.

4. Mashed Squash Salad

Calories: 90 kcal| Total time: 10 minutes| Servings: 6|Difficulty: Easy

Ingredients:

- Allspice, 1 teaspoon.

- Blue Agave, ¼ cup, natural

- Squash 2, skinned & cubed

- Sea Salt, 1/8 teaspoon.

- Date Sugar, ¼ cup

- Hemp Milk, ¼ cup

Directions

1. Put the squash chunks and the water in a saucepan over medium flame.

2. Boil the mixture and simmer for twenty minutes or when the squash is soft.

3. When soft, drain the water, then mash the squash.

4. After this, add a spoon of date sugar, organic milk, spice, sea salt and agave. Mix it well.

5. Serve yourself and love it.

5. Chickpeas Salad

Calories: 558 kcal| Total time: 40 minutes| Servings: 4|Difficulty: Easy

Ingredients:

- Chickpeas, 1 ½ cups, washed

- Red onion, ½ cup, cubed

- Cilantro, ¼ cup, fresh one & well chopped

- Avocado, 1 cup

- Sea salt as per taste

Directions

1. First, put the chickpeas in a bowl and mash it with the masher.

2. Add the avocado and then mix it properly.

3. In this mixture, add lemon juice and blend properly. Then whisk with the lime juice, blend, and mix with the cilantro. Stir it again. Then, add a spoon of salt. Whisk it again.

4. Serve and enjoy yourself

6. Fetish Mango Salad

Calories: 558 kcal| Total time: 45 minutes| Servings: 4|Difficulty: Easy

Ingredients:

- Mangoes, 2

- Red onion, 1/4

- Cherry tomatoes, 1/4 cup

- Cucumber 1/2, having seeds

- Bell pepper ½, green

- Key lime, 1

- Sea salt according to taste

- Cayenne pepper according to taste

Directions: Preparing Mango Salad begins with cutting the mangoes, chopping the red onion, and slicing the cherry tomatoes. Slice thinly the seeded cucumber as well as the bell pepper. In a little tub, add all the ingredients and mix. Take the lime and spill over the salad.

Sprinkle with salt and cayenne pepper and leave for marinating in the refrigerator for about 20 minutes before feeding. Enjoy it as your salad, salsa or even a dip; that is your call!

7. Kidney friendly Strawberry and dandelion Salad

Calories: 250 kcal| Total time: 50 minutes| Servings: 4|Difficulty: Easy

Ingredients:

- Grape-seed oil, 2 tablespoons

- Strawberries, 10, chopped

- Red onion, 1 medium, chopped

- Dandelion greens, 4 cups

- Key lime juice, 2 tablespoons

- Sea salt as per taste

Directions:

1. Take a nonstick pan, put grape-seed oil in it, heat it over medium flame. Add sea salt and the sliced onions to the pan. Cook and stir regularly until the onions are smooth, softly golden.

2. In a cup, add lime juice to the strawberry slices.

3. Clean the dandelion greens and break them into bite-sized bits.

4. Once the onions are almost done, pour the rest of the key lime juice into the pan, then cook for a few minutes till the onions are browned.

5. Remove from heat. In the salad bowl, mix the onions, greens, and strawberries along with all of the juices. Sprinkle the sea salt.

6. Serve and enjoy.

8. Grilled Vegetable Pasta Salad

Calories: 377 kcal| Total time: 50 minutes| Servings: 8|Difficulty: Easy

Ingredients

- Garlic cloves, minced, 2

- Gijon mustard, 1 tablespoon

- Lemon juice, 1/4 cup)

- Olive oil, 1/4 cup

- Black pepper, 1/2 teaspoon

- Rotini, uncooked, 12 ounces

- Zucchini, sliced, 2 meds

- Head anise, sliced, 1

- Quartered mushrooms, 8

- Red onion, sliced, 1 med

- Fresh basil leaves, shredded, 2 tablespoons

- Fresh thyme, 1 tablespoon

- Fresh parsley, chopped, 1 tablespoon

Instructions

1. Make the dressing by adding all the ingredients in a mixing bowl together and whisking them together,

2. All vegetables are added to a big mixing bowl. Pour half of the dressing over the vegetables and mix until they are all finely coated. Allow the vegetables to marinate when cooking the pasta according to the package directions. In cool water, rinse the noodles.

3. Turn the oven on to broil in the meantime or start cooking up the barbeque. If the oven is used, use the greased broiler pan, or use the grill basket if using the barbeque.

4. Spread the vegetables on the broiling pan or the hot grill basket the vegetable mixture and cook until the vegetables become golden brown. To allow the browning to occur uniformly, stir them after every 4-5 mins. Pour in a serving bowl when browned, add the pasta & the leftover dressing, and add the fresh herbs. Toss, then serve.

Chapter 7: Kidney Friendly Renal Diet Snacks

1. Homemade renal friendly sausage

Calories: 93 kcal| Total time: 25 minutes| Servings: 8|Difficulty: Medium

Ingredients

- Onion, 1⁄2 cup, finely chopped

- Olive oil, 2 tablespoons

- Dried sage, 2 teaspoons

- Fresh ground 1 teaspoon, black pepper

- Sugar, 1 tablespoon

- Red pepper flakes, 1⁄8 teaspoon

- Ground cloves, 1 pinch

- Fresh thyme, 1 teaspoon, finely chopped.

- Egg yolk, 1 large

- Lean pork, 2 lbs. ground

Directions

1. Cook onion in olive oil on moderately low heat till soft and brown. Cool them for 10 minutes.

2. Combine sage, pepper, sugar, thyme, and cloves in a bowl.

3. Place egg yolk, reserved onion and pork in a large bowl and add mixed spices.

4. Make 16 patties.

5. Pan fry them in a large skillet for 5 minutes on both sides.

6. Serve.

2. Kidney friendly fruit dip

Calories: 123 kcal| Total time: 20 minutes| Servings: 10|Difficulty: Easy

Ingredients

- Sour Cream, 1 Cup, (Low phosphorous dip)

- Brown Sugar, 2 Tablespoon

- Vanilla Extract, 1/2 Teaspoon

Instructions

1. Mix brown sugar, sour cream, and vanilla extract.

2. Let it stand in a refrigerator for the flavors to combine (at least 1 hr. or 2 hr. or better overnight).

3. Cut all fruits such as bananas, grapes, apples, melon, oranges, strawberries, peaches, pears, or watermelon into chunks or as desired.

4. To prevent discoloration, Dip apples, bananas in some lemon juice.

5. Place the fruit at the edge of serving dish.

6. Place the dip in dish in enter of tray.

3. Heavenly Deviled Eggs

Calories: 98 kcal| Total time: 10 minutes| Servings: 4|Difficulty: Easy

Ingredients

- Eggs, hard boiled, shells removed, 4 large

- Light mayonnaise, 2 tablespoons

- Dry mustard, ½ teaspoon

- Cider vinegar, ½ teaspoon

- Onion, finely chopped, 1 tablespoon

- Ground black pepper, ¼ teaspoon

- Dash of paprika, optional garnish

Directions

1. Cut the eggs into half, lengthwise. Now carefully remove the yolks and

   place them in small bowl. Transfer egg white in a plate.

2. Mix yolks with the help of fork and add vinegar, onion, dry mustard, and black pepper.

3. Now refill the egg white with the yolk mixture, piling slightly.

4. Finally sprinkle the deviled eggs with some paprika.

5. Serve.

4. Sweet & Nutty Protein Bars

Calories: 283 kcal| Total time: 30 minutes| Servings: 8|Difficulty: Easy

Ingredients

- Rolled oats, toasted, 2½ cups

- Almonds, ½ cup

- Flaxseeds, ½ cup

- Peanut butter, ½ cup

- Dried cherries, 1 cup, blueberries or craisins®

- Honey, ½ cup

Instructions

1. Toast the oats by placing rolled oats on a baking sheet in a 350° F oven for 10 minutes or until golden brown.

2. Mix all ingredients together until well-mixed.

3. Press the protein mix down into a lightly greased 9" x 9" pan. Wrap and refrigerate for at least one hour or overnight.

4. Cut protein bars into desired squares then serve.

5. Crispy Cauliflower Phyllo Cups

Calories: 283 kcal| Total time: 30 minutes| Servings: 8|Difficulty: Easy

Ingredients

- Beaten, lightly scrambled, 3 eggs

- Swiss cheese, ½ cup, shredded

- Cheddar cheese, ½ cup, shredded

- Butter, 2 tablespoons

- Natural and uncured, 4 slices bacon, diced

- Cauliflower, diced, cooked, 1½ cups

- Onions, finely diced, ¼ cup

- Jalapeños, diced, 2 tablespoons

- Red pepper flakes, ½ teaspoon

- Parsley, 1 tablespoon

- Ground black pepper, ½ teaspoon

- Phyllo dough, 3 sheets

- Parsley, black pepper, optional garnish

Instructions

1. Preheat the oven to 375° F.

2. In a large pan, scramble the eggs, then remove them and set aside.

3. In same pan, melt the butter and sauté bacon till cooked. Add onions, jalapeños, cauliflower, and red pepper, sauté till the onions become translucent. Now season with ground black pepper parsley.

4. Then remove from the heat and add scrambled eggs and two cheeses.

5. Now layer three phyllo sheets and cut the sheets in 24 squares, press lightly on mini muffin tin pan.

6. Now fill each cup with same amounts of mix, bake on bottom shelf of oven for almost 12 to 15 minutes, or till slightly golden. Turn off the oven and let them rest for almost 2–3 minutes.

7. Serve.

6. Kidney friendly Orange and Cinnamon Biscotti

Calories: 273 kcal| Total time: 1 hr. 8 minutes| Servings: 8|Difficulty: Easy

Ingredients

- Sugar, 1 cup

- Unsalted butter, room temperature, ½ cup

- Eggs, 2 large

- Grated orange peel, 2 teaspoons

- Vanilla extract, 1 teaspoon

- All-purpose flour, 2 cups

- Cream of tartar, 1 teaspoon

- Baking soda, ½ teaspoon

- Ground cinnamon, 1 teaspoon

- Salt, ¼ teaspoon

Instructions

1. Preheat the oven to 325° F.

2. Spray two baking sheets using nonstick cooking spray.

3. Beat the sugar & unsalted butter in large bowl till well blended.

4. Now add eggs 1 at a time, beat well after each.

5. Add in orange peel & vanilla.

6. Now mix flour, baking soda, cream of tartar, cinnamon, and salt.

7. Then add dry ingredients to the butter mixture and then mix until completely incorporated.

8. Now divide the dough in half. Put each half in a sheet. With floured hands, make each half to log shape which is three inches wide by 3 quarters of the inch high. Then bake till the dough logs become firm to touch, around 35 minutes.

9. Now remove the dough logs from the oven and cool them for 10 minutes.

10. Then transfer the logs to a surface. By using knife, cut ½-inch-thick slices in diagonal. Arrange the cut side down on the baking sheets.

11. Now bake till the bottoms turns golden, around 12 minutes.

12. Flip biscotti over; then bake till bottoms are golden, around 12 minutes longer.

13. Take out from the wire rack, cool

14. Serve.

Conclusion

For chronic kidney disease, there is currently no proven treatment, but there are habits and activities that can reduce the progression of kidney failure, including lifestyle behaviors. For those who have diabetes, heart disease, high blood pressure, or have a history of kidney failure, they are already at risk for kidney disease. And this book I've dedicated it precisely to people who want to change their nutritional style, learn how to quickly and easily cook healthy, light foods that can relieve your kidneys.

All the recipes are designed for beginners in the kitchen and I hope you enjoyed them a lot. Continue on this path, there are no definitive cures but with perseverance and patience we can succeed together to feed ourselves better, try and try again these recipes and stay healthy as much as possible. Thank you so much for your trust and I hope you will continue to follow me with the next quick and easy cookbooks.

I wish you all the best

CPSIA information can be obtained
at www.ICGtesting.com
Printed in the USA
BVHW041156090321
602109BV00016B/327

9 781801 540353